Lifting the Lid

mandy duggan

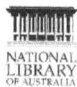

Copyright © 2020 Mandy Duggan
All rights reserved.
ISBN-13   978-1-922343-53-6

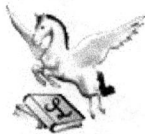

Linellen Press
265 Boomerang Road
Oldbury, Western Australia
www.linellenpress.com.au

Dedication

With gratitude to the loves of my life, my children, Neesha and Josh. For inspiring me to always live my best life.

.

Will you sit with me when I hit the wall; will you wrap your arms around me in my darkest moment to let me know that I am not alone?

Will you truly be with me because you know that I need you to be; because you know that you would not want to be alone in your darkest moment?

Do you hear the rhythm of life and the beat of the ocean tide? Do you smile at early morning birdsong? Do you rejoice in the sound of children's laughter?

Can you be still and listen to the wind. Can you watch the sky without looking at your watch? Can you be fully present in every moment?

Will you walk in the garden and close your eyes to appreciate the fragrance of the frangipani blossom? Does that speak directly to your senses?

Do you glory in the feel of the sun on your face? Does this give you hope and an urge to dance? Does the beauty of the sunrise stop your mind?

Can you feel your heartbeat when your fingers are entwined in mine; does this give you the sense that you are home?

Do you long for that moment when there is only your heartbeat and mine and you know you have found your other half?

Can you hear me calling for you in the silence; will you come to me without thinking about what time you must get up for work?

Are you mesmerised by the curve of my neck and the smile in my eyes? Do you see the bee on the rosebud as a wondrous thing?

Can you see the future and the past when you look into my eyes? Can you see my mood in the way that I hold my shoulders?

Would you be willing to go against what is right for you to be my friend or will you always stay true to your values and beliefs even if that means hurting my feelings?

Can I share with you my deepest secrets and fears and know that you won't use them against me?

Will you intuitively know that when I love someone I give a piece of myself to them to take as their own? And when someone I love dies, that piece of me dies with them?

Will you lead me to the sunshine if I am living in the shade? Will you encourage me to abandon the limits that I place on myself, to lift the lid so that I can be the best version of me?

This journey within knows no bounds.

I used to wonder if I would reach the end of my self-discovery, an *are we there yet?!* mentality. Now, I give that no thought and just dive right in.

What I am learning continually is that I do not begin and I do not end. There is no limit to what I can achieve, unless I limit myself.

I have faced situations that I thought would be unbearable to me; that I could not comprehend, that caused my mind to scream *Nooooo!*

And the only sensible thing that I could do to help myself through these situations was to dive within. I really underestimated my ability to cope. I learned that I am so much stronger and courageous than I thought possible.

The morning is unfolding beautifully for me; I am absorbed in the view from my window, the sound of the birds outside and the beauty of my roses abuzz with bees. There's a gentle breeze, and foliage flutters in sync with the touch of the breeze on my skin as it wafts through the open window. In this moment, I am completely present and at peace.

Not a thought about what I ought to be doing or what needs to be done. Just pure alignment of energy and silence in my mind. Domestic violence; heartache; poverty; hunger and famine; child sex trade; Isis and terrorism; and human suffering seem like they belong to another life; another world.

Do you have moments like these?

These are moments we tend to not recognise as beautiful, that we tend to not commit to memory; moments we tend to not share with each other, almost as if because they fill our hearts, they are not worthy of conversation.

I worked on my book yesterday, editing *William Absolutely Uninvited*. My right eye cried the whole time. If you have read that book, you will understand. When I went to bed, I was emotionally churning.

Last night was one of broken sleep and vivid dreams and I alternated my pillow from one end of the bed to the other. I often do this when I am unable to sleep. But, with the hum of the ceiling fan soothing me, I managed to drift off.

Words kept coming to me while I was sleeping and when I woke this morning, I knew it was time to begin. It was time to lift the lid.

Lifting the Lid is two-fold for me.

It is *no longer* suppressing past trauma, joy or love. It is *no longer* suppressing that which makes me feel uncomfortable. It is working through pain and fear and anger – *no longer* containing it within my mind and my body. No shutting the lid on anything, to either contain or hide what needs to be acknowledged and loved.

It is also not giving in to my insecurities and limiting my life because of them. It is choosing to live without the limitations that I place on myself both because of past trauma and belief systems that no longer serve me. It is believing and embracing that I can have the life that is intended for me, if I just allow myself to. It is taking away the ceiling that I place on my dreams and ambitions.

Since 2014, I have been climbing a mountain and I am now sitting quietly at the top – or perhaps it is just a ledge and there is more climbing to be done. Following a diagnosis of a rare and incurable type of blood cancer in 2014, my journey within helped me to accept that the cancer is a part of myself (and not some rotten, unwelcome third party) and to truly know myself and understand the emotions raging inside of me.

This is a journey I will always be on. I call it *life*. Rather than focus on the cancer, I choose to focus on living my best life in every moment.

To do this, I am committed to my own truth. Authentic is the only way to live my best life, my thoughts, feelings and actions in perfect alignment. I am very in tune with my body and am quick to recognise the dis-ease that I feel when I do not come from my truth and am not authentic. I have no doubt that years of dis-ease and going against what is right for me to avoid conflict and trauma have contributed to my current health.

I am committed to being there for myself one hundred percent.

Always.

Just thinking that makes me tingle and smile.

I am committed to saying those things that I used to swallow back down before they could be spoken.

I am committed to keeping my heart wide open even at the most painful times.

I am committed to always coming from love despite my conditioning to come from anger or fear or shame.

The journey has been epic so far, full of struggle and self-discovery and yet so rewarding in many ways.

Will you sit with me when I hit the wall; will you wrap your arms around me in my darkest moment to let me know that I am not alone?

I have been assessing what is important to me. I am always doing this. Always coming from the sense of who I am and how I fit in to this world; how my energy aligns and the impact that I have. This is the only way to know myself.

My journey of healing requires acknowledgement of what has hurt me in the past; what brings me joy and what matters right now, in this moment. This acknowledgement also reveals to me who I am. This requires absolute honesty, which has been such a challenge as I have discovered that I have often been dishonest, downplaying a situation or emotion so that I can be okay with what is happening when I am actually not okay with it.

I have been gathering these things that are important to me like jewels and keeping them in a burgundy velvet bag, with a gold, tasseled draw string at the top.

I used to think that I was defined by what I did; how I filled my time. Actually, I did not just think it, there was no separation between what I did and who I was, like those things were my identity.

Almost every introduction to someone I hadn't met before began with them asking "what do you do for work?" I was guilty of asking the same thing of others, many times. I lived that way for a long time.

I no longer live that way.

When I was no longer able to work due to poor health, I began to dread meeting new people. I dreaded being asked what I do. I felt that I had nothing of myself to offer the person asking, because I no longer went to a place of employment. It was as if I was nobody, like I no longer existed.

Effectively I did nothing. Well nothing that I thought would be understood or valued by anyone else, which made me realise that I did not value myself if I was not working. I felt that I was a failure because I could not work. I also felt angry that the person asking had no interest in what I was passionate about, what brought me to life. I talked to my therapist about this issue and was able to recognise what I do each day. I was able to recognise what my purpose is.

This started a change in the way I thought about myself. I became intrigued to discover me. I became aware of how precious this opportunity was for me to discover myself. To learn who I truly am inside all those layers of conditioning and beliefs that were long outdated and no longer serving me.

What a magical journey I embarked on. An all roads lead to Mandy journey.

Now, when I am asked, "what do you do?" my response is *"I invest in my health and well-being, I am 100% committed to self-care"*.

What a wonderful and empowering response that is, not just for me, but also for the person asking. Don't you think?

I now look forward to meeting new people and being asked "what do you do?"

What matters to me is connection, not conversation, connection. Without connection, conversation is meaningless.

What is most important is that I no longer abandon myself, not for someone else's ideals or demands or because I do not understand my own needs and my own truth.

I appreciate my own need to remain true to my beliefs and values and I appreciate that we each have the same need for authenticity.

I am stepping away from people in my life who do not align with this belief. Co-dependency is rife, with people living a fake life and requiring that you accept this fakeness to keep friendships; to keep relationships. It is so easy to be co-dependent. To give in to someone else's expectations of you. To keep the peace rather than speak one's truth. To make excuses for poor choices and behaviour because it makes another person happy; regardless that you abandon yourself in the process.

Co-dependency was vital to my existence as a child who grew up in a home that was rife with alcohol abuse, post-traumatic stress disorder, rage, violence and chaos. I became an expert at gauging how I needed to act in order to keep myself safe and to avoid setting off a proverbial hand grenade.

I aim to no longer do this. Some people have moved out of my life because of this. I am okay with this – I accept that it has needed to happen so that I am able to truly be who I am always.

How amazing it feels to not abandon myself, to remain in my truth at all times.

Who am I, if I am not myself? Indeed.

Connection to self. I rarely listened to my inner wisdom, mostly because I was not connected with myself.

When I was a child, it was necessary for me to disconnect with myself to survive the trauma of abuse. I was alive and life was happening to me. I was not making things happen for me. I was surviving; nothing more.

There is a very tangible difference between life happening and making life happen.

As I began to know myself, in the years of recovery from diagnosis of a chronic disease and severe anxiety, I began to listen in the stillness and know what is right for me. I began to know that I have the answers to the questions and that all I need to do is be still and listen to the silence. Because in stillness and silence I could see my own truth.

I began to have faith that I would know what I needed to do in any given situation. I would know when I was aligned with my thoughts and my actions.

I am learning to be present and open-hearted, to be there for myself in my darkest times and in my times of fearfulness.

I am learning to fully embrace the times

when my heart is completely aligned with my purpose and I am at peace. I am learning just how precious that really is.

I am beginning to understand how necessary that is to me; to understand how vital it is to remain present, to be with myself at all times. I am no longer retreating to a dark place where I barely breathe and I am paralysed with fear or I am numb.

As a child, I experienced significant trauma associated with verbal abuse, physical abuse and sexual abuse. I became adept at disconnecting with myself at a young age and honed this skill throughout my life. This was a valuable skill for me, especially during my younger years when I was living with abuse every day and at the complete mercy of the people who abused me.

To unlearn this, to try to stay present when I would usually dissociate, is an ongoing process for me. However, I work hard at staying present and am more aware of when I am not. There are times when I disassociate because I cannot emotionally cope and I need to slip into almost a third person mode. Take a step back from what is happening, so I can cope. I will continue to change this so I can stay present, I am committed to this.

In December 2019, I began treatment for blood cancer. I arrived at a place I did not want to be. Yet I knew that I must be at this place. With so much going on, I didn't have the luxury of time; time to be with myself for as long as it took. It would have been so easy to dissociate and disconnect from the thoughts and fear and slip into auto pilot. A lot easier than sitting with myself for as long as it took.

But sit with myself I did. Reassuring myself, that while I may not want to be at this place, I am here and I want to have life and therefore I choose to have this treatment. And sit with myself, I continue to do. As I write this chapter, I am 4 cycles into a 6 cycle (each cycle is 28 days) treatment regime and with each cycle, I have been able to support myself on a deeper level. There were many days that I suffered acute nausea and vomiting and all I could do was to lay on my bed, underneath the ceiling fan, with a bucket beside my bed. The only person who could get me through these times, was me. I discovered a depth to myself that I never knew I had and I never left myself, not even for a moment.

I know that I can sit with myself, when I hit the wall. I am discovering that there are others that will sit me with too.

Connection to another. Connection to women has not been overly difficult for me; I cherish the way women care about each other and hold space for each other. Although, I have had periods of time in my life, where I could not have connection with my mother. I believe wholeheartedly that my mother did the best that she could at the time, yet she did not protect me from abuse and I felt very abandoned. The impact of trauma on my life is significant and there were times when I was furious with my mother and could not be around her. I am more aware now of the triggers when I am around my mother and I am able to be fully present and open-hearted when I am with her. As she becomes older and frailer, I cherish every moment that I am able to spend with her, aware of how special it is that I am now able to absorb the wonderful experience of holding her hand or just sitting with her.

Connection to men has been the complete opposite for me. Childhood exposure to a violent, alcoholic and angry father and sexual abuse by several men outside my family, bred fear of men and I did not want to connect to men or to myself when I was being abused.

I became quite fragmented because of the abuse that I suffered as a child. When I was no longer a child, I was attracted to men who did not show me kindness or friendship. I was attracted to men who were verbally abusive and angry, men that I ultimately moved away from and that left me feeling unworthy and unlovable.

In recent months I have been focused on improving my connection with men and increasing my connection with women.

I no longer avoid what makes me feel unworthy and afraid; I now choose to invite those things in and sit with myself through the shame and fear and whatever comes up for me. Hey, I squirm, and I am uncomfortable, but I do not abandon myself.

I am also learning that connection to another does not require disconnection from self.

I have spent a significant chunk of my life putting my own needs behind those of another person. This automatically disconnects me from myself. I no longer do this; I realise how fundamentally important it is for me to never compromise my values and beliefs.

In all of my intimate relationships, with the type of men that I chose, I found myself totally unsupported when I hit the wall. In fact, in my marriage, I was ridiculed for it. I wasn't able to sit with myself and the men in my life would not sit with me either.

My relationship with myself was so poor I thought I was deserving of this treatment. I did not think I was worthy of anything more at the time.

More recently, I have an expectation with my close relationships that I will remain authentic and true to myself at all times. This is something I would always say was a value that I sought out in others. Yet, I compromised this value for myself. Every time. With every relationship.

I could not speak my truth for fear I would be rejected if my truth was not aligned with that of another person – also, for fear that it would not be safe to be true to myself.

Standing firmly in my truth can be a lonely place, yet this is how I sit with myself. Staying true to myself. I show up every time.

I have learned there is nothing I am not able to work through, if I do not abandon myself. I am able to accept situations rather than resist them with all my might.

Connection to nature. I spend a lot of time in nature, even if that means sitting in my back yard, among the trees, with the birds and the breeze.

When I become extremely anxious, I take off my shoes and sit on the lawn, with my bare feet connecting with the earth and I watch the sky between the branches and leaves of the trees. I walk in my garden and smell the fragrance of the flowers and I spend time watching the bees and the butterflies.

I never had time for this before, or the inclination. I never made time for this. I used to think that spending time in nature was for hippies. I used to rush through life and barely see nature around me. I was far too busy for such nonsense.

Not now.

At the moment I am staying on a property in Jilliby, New South Wales, with my sister. Twenty-five acres of land, some cleared and paddocked and some uncleared, with trees. It is my idea of paradise. There are resident wallabies often in full view, nibbling on the lawn. It doesn't matter how many times I see a wallaby I am still delighted every time. The birdsong is the most beautiful of sounds and completely in tune with the surroundings.

My bedroom looks out on this view and

when I first open my eyes, it takes my breath away. Every time.

Connection to the ocean. Arguably, the ocean is nature. Yet, it really does deserve its own category because by soul definition it is vastly different to hugging a tree or bush walking. Time by the ocean has helped me to ground many times, when nothing else could.

These past six years, in particular, I have spent many hours by the ocean. However, I have always found solace at the beach. Walking, sitting, and laying. Always with my feet in the sand. Sometimes with my feet in the water. Always with the sun on my face.

I am not a keen swimmer in the ocean. A childhood near-drowning incident traumatised me greatly and the residual memory of that prevents me from feeling uninhibited when I am submerged in the ocean.

Yet, I crave and often seek the solace of being by the ocean. I connect with the flow and ebb of the tide and liken it to my own endurance to continue to breathe in and out, no matter what is going on around me, in my life.

Similarly, the ocean continues to ebb and flow, no matter what is happening in the world. It is something I can be certain of, in a very uncertain world. Certainty in an unpredictable environment such as *life* is an anchor for my anxious mind.

Will you truly be with me because you know that I need you to be; because you know that you would not want to be alone in your darkest moment? With no thought for how much I earn?

Everywhere, people seem to be caught up in *doing*, to such an extent that most do not know how to *be*. Or most do not know that there is a vast difference between *doing* and *being*.

I see the sacrifice that some people make blindly, every moment of every day. (That is not a criticism, it's an observation.) I see the disconnection from self. Everywhere. I recognise myself in them.

It touches a place of great sorrow deep inside my soul to see so many people on this particular mouse wheel, to see so many people who have lost touch with what is important or perhaps have never been in touch with what is important. The disconnection is necessary so that people can continue to live this type of existence.

Collection of material things does not bring

happiness – the kind of happiness that radiates out of you. If that is your highest priority, it requires disconnection and emptiness. Things do not resonate with our soul, moments do. I am not saying that you must be without material things to have happiness. It is more about the attachment that one has to material things and whether they value this more than human connection and connection with self.

As people continue to put work and earning money as their highest priority thinking that this is what will fulfil them – the more people believe that the amount of money they earn, the level of access they have to material things – defines them, that it somehow makes them more powerful, more successful or more significant than another.

Take this further and people start to choose their friends, the people they want to be seen with based on how much money their friends earn and the status they associate with being seen with those people.

Once you have a profound connection with yourself and live out of your truth, it is difficult to be around people who are not living with this level of self-awareness.

To me, this class system seems such an

empty existence. A fear-based existence. Without meaning.

As people put themselves under unbelievable pressure to keep up with the Jones's they become even more disconnected to their souls and the calling of what is needed for their happiness; the calling for fulfilment; the calling for authenticity.

When faced with moments where you find yourself fighting for life, everything falls away and there is just you in the room and your soul. Nothing more. And you realise what is truly important.

How grand the roof is over your head and how flash your car is has no bearing on this. None.

It is very much about taking the next breath. It is about digging deep inside yourself and discovering the strength to endure and to get up and live.

I live with a meagre income from a Disability Support Pension. Prior to this, I lived a frugal life as a sole parent, supplementing welfare with income from part-time work, followed by three and a half years of receiving New Start Allowance ($34.00 a day) while I made numerous applications to Centrelink for

Disability Support Pension and numerous appeals. This existence gave me the insight into what is really important. It gave me insight into what my values were and what values I wanted to pass onto my children.

To me, wealth has nothing to do with money. Money is something that is needed to provide food and shelter.

To me wealth is enrichment, not of the money kind, the enrichment of love of self, the love of your family, the respect and loyalty of your friends: the moments that take your breath away.

Wealth is aspiring to leave a person better than when you found them. Wealth is giving to another in need, with no expectation other than to connect with your purpose. Wealth is knowing you have made a difference to someone's life.

I would rather not have a friend, a lover or an acquaintance if those relationships were based on how much money I earn or how much money the people I know earn. I no longer live a fake existence, a life based on measuring myself against money or material possessions.

I no longer spend time with people who seek out material worth in a person over whether that person has a kind heart and authenticity.

I believe the people who live in my heart do so because we share a common bond. We see each other. We see the beauty of each other's heart. We see each other's integrity. We know we can call upon one another in our darkest moment, should we not want to be alone. We will show up for one another.

Those people that I can be with when I am at my worst as well as at my best and know that there is no judgment are the ones I keep close always.

They are the people I hold space for; the people I pray for without them knowing. They are among my greatest treasures.

It is not easy to be with myself in my darkest moments. My instinct has always been to disconnect, to seek distraction and suppress the darkness. As I seek to love all parts of myself, including the darkness, I am committed to staying present when I feel shame in my belly or sadness in my heart, or anger, or grief.

Sometimes I disconnect still … more than I would like.

Unbecoming what I have been for so long takes time – perhaps my entire lifetime – and it takes self-compassion and such courage.

I am not a visual person. I am an energy person. I sense. I often sense the pain of another person and my first instinct is to want to wrap my arms around that person and comfort them.

I am committed to offering myself this comfort too.

Do you hear the rhythm of life and the beat of the ocean tide? Do you smile at early morning birdsong? Do you rejoice in the sound of children's laughter?

We all love music in one way or another, right? We have connection with lyrics and tunes that remind us of happy times and sad times? I know that I do.

Music has been prevalent in my life.

Both of my parents could belt out a tune and stop the room. I have fond memories of my dad singing *Danny Boy* and it was a must for his funeral service.

It turned out that so could I. I would sing at many events, sometimes pre-arranged, but more often someone else would arrange for me to sing and I did not know about it until I was being invited to the stage.

I recall the record player and The Everley Brothers, Elvis and Roy Orbison, amongst others. Music is a real trip down memory lane for me.

I have a guitar which I do not pick up often enough and my fingers are always painful on the steel strings yet, when I'm in the mood, strumming my guitar and singing is one of my happy places.

Music touches everyone in one way or another. Some people have multiple playlists of music in their phones, some pay for Spotify, blue-toothing tunes through their speakers, tapping their feet, moving their hips as they get on with their day.

Some still listen to their radio or play a CD.

I have a collection of cassette tapes that I treasure. I can no longer play them as I don't have a cassette player, yet I cannot bring myself to discard them.

I love a good dance too. Music has been and continues to be a large part of my life, including playing my guitar, singing, playing my hapi drum and going to music events. A particular treasure is my clear quartz crystal singing bowl.

For therapy, I regularly attend a live harp session and also sound journeys with sound bowls and gonging. These are amazing, beyond words and if you haven't experienced music therapies, you are not living fully!

For five years I was part of a band and I

wrote my own songs. This was an amazing part of my life, full of creative expression. I was a singer in the three-piece band, with acoustic guitar accompaniment, performing our original material.

I recall a conversation with someone I met many years ago. I asked what his favourite song was and he shared the name of the song and the artist – this conversation was actually an electronic exchange of words. I remember listening to that song on Youtube: *I fooled around and fell in love*. It's about a man who was not loyal to one woman, treated them like conquests, until he fell in love. I wondered what it was about this song that made it a favourite. I had thoughts of a teenage boy who believed his mother had abandoned him. He was being raised by his father; perhaps this was the music his father played and without a thought for the lyrics, this became his favourite song because it reminded him of a time in his life.

This conversation struck a deep chord in me at the time. It was thought-provoking. The different ways each of us relates to music and what part it plays in our life.

Me? I love a good solo, award-winning performance in the shower or while I'm cleaning house.

I am listening to Spotify while I write at the moment. Vincent (starry, starry night) is playing. Such a beautiful and haunting song. Deeply moving. I sense the suffering of Vincent, his pain, his vulnerability.

What I really want to talk about is the music and rhythm that so many of us do not hear. The magical sounds that happen around us every moment of every day that so many of us are completely tuned out to.

The peppermint trees in my back yard attract many birds. I can hear birdsong any time on any given day. I delight in this, absolutely. It is truly magical. Yet some people are annoyed by this music and think of it as noise.

I sometimes use this birdsong as an opportunity for mindfulness, to be completely in the moment. Just me and the birdsong. No thoughts of what needs to be done, what I should have done or what else I ought to be doing with this time. Other times, I simply enjoy the sounds.

I relish in the fact that I am giving myself the gift of *being*.

I recall the sunsets in spring and summer and the cicada orchestra that entertains me while I water my roses. The sound resonates with my heart and my emotions, touches my soul. I am completely aligned in these moments. Serene.

My home is in close proximity to the ocean and on a still night I can hear the waves crashing. I do not need to leave my home to hear the ocean. I am truly blessed.

As I write this chapter, I am at sea on a very large cruise ship and I have been spending time out on deck or by the windows, with views of the ocean as far as I can see. Being here has clarified for me how much the sounds of the ocean resonate with me. Cruising on the ocean, the sounds of the flow and ebb of the waves are absent and I miss these.

Among my favourite music is that of children laughing. It is infectious! I have a huge collection in the closets of my mind of my children laughing with me, with each other, with their friends, when they were young and carefree.

We still laugh together, with each other and at each other, my children and I. They are adults now so the music is a different tone and depth, but goodness; it fills my heart with joy.

My neighbour of many years, moved out of the house next door a couple of years ago, with her two children. I used to love the sound of her children playing and laughing in the back yard. This sound gives me hope. Now, I hear silence from this backyard and the absence of this music is poignant.

Can you be still and listen to the wind? Can you watch the sky without looking at your watch? Can you be fully present in every moment?

What is it you do to fill you days? Do you cram in things so you just do not stop, so there is no time for thoughts? No time for feelings?

Do you ignore the calling of your soul, because you are just too busy to listen? Do you hear the calling of your soul?

Are you so disconnected from yourself that you have no idea that illness or uneasy feelings may just be messages from your soul, to pay attention?

So many of us are disconnected from ourselves with no awareness of this state. My mind reflects on addiction, the things we fill our lives with to avoid emotional pain and suffering.

Addictions: the things that people do repetitively to avoid feeling emotional pain. The things that must be done, no matter what else needs to be done, whether they are good for you or not. I believe emphatically that addiction arises out of emotional pain. I believe that addiction is the discovery of something that eases, distracts one from, or numbs emotional pain and the craving to continue to do this something repeatedly, rather than feel.

Addiction takes many forms: physical activity, work, substance abuse – drugs (prescription and illicit), alcohol, tobacco, retail therapy, eating, chewing fingernails, sex, gambling, twirling your hair in your fingers … the list goes on.

I do not want to know what you do to avoid emotional pain. I do not want to know what you fill your life with to avoid the stillness that gives you time to feel and to know yourself completely.

What I do want to know is whether you can be with yourself; whether you can be there for yourself to process your feelings and understand the message they are trying to say to you; whether you can hear your soul's calling; that you will refrain from addictive and distractive behaviour and stay with yourself and how you are feeling; that you will stop doing and just be; whether you can be with yourself for as long as it takes.

I have learned how valuable it is to be still; to hear the wind and let that sound resonate with my soul. How necessary that is, for me.

And for you.

My dear friend recently arranged to meet a friend while travelling in New Zealand. It had been more than 12 months since they caught up, neither knowing when they would cross paths in the future. Her friend allotted three hours to catch up and spent the whole time checking his watch, leaving dot on the time he had allocated.

She talked about how this made her feel, this continual checking of the watch. Her pain spilled out of her eyes and down her face as she talked about this.

What does this say to you? What thoughts does it provoke?

Will you adjust your schedule to do what is needed?

It really is not a nice feeling when someone is with you but not fully present. It certainly feeds into low self-esteem.

Will you take off your shoes just to feel the earth beneath your feet? – without thought of the time it will take to remove your socks and shoes and put them back on again? – without thinking that your feet may get dirty? Valuing and recognising how vital it is for your feet to connect with the earth, skin on sand, above the passage of time.

I used to walk along the ocean front every day, shoes and socks on, pounding the pavement with spectacular views of the ocean the whole way. I contemplated walking on the sand but the thought of taking my shoes off and having to carry them then clean off the sand to put them back on was enough to stop me from doing it. For years I did that walk.

Then one day, I decided to just take my shoes off and walk on the beach, sand in my toes. The thoughts of time and inconvenience were politely told to be quiet. I no longer deny myself that pleasure and take all the time I need to walk on the beach.

I often recommend laying outdoors and looking at the sky to friends or family when they talk to me about feeling stressed or anxious. This is something that really helps me when I am anxious and stressed and brings me into the 'now' quickly. I am often asked *"how long do I need to do this for?"* For as long as it takes.

I have days that start with weariness, low brain function; days which require that I just be.

These may be part days, consecutive days, even weeks. I am becoming better at being there, with myself, for as long as it takes.

No questioning why I am feeling this way — did I get enough sleep? Did I overdo things? Has something happened to make me feel flat? Just acceptance, self-love, staying present and having my own back.

I spent years ignoring my body, my energy levels and my health —

— years of existing without regard for what I needed, and fitting into a society that shouts the *Soldier on!* message loud and clear

— years of spending my days doing what was expected of me: going to work, being a parent, being a wife, being a friend, even when I was tired or unwell

— years of catching the cold that your co-worker spread throughout the workplace because they, too, ignored what their body needed

— years of catching the gastro that went around and only staying home until the vomiting or diarrhea had passed with no thought for contagions or the need for the body to recover

— years of feeling the stress and pressure to

return to work when my child was at home with chicken pox and could not attend school until it was no longer contagious, and I needed to be at home with them

— years of not being fully present because I was thinking about where else I needed to be, frustrated at this child for being sick, annoyed because my workplace made demands on me at a time when I needed to be with my child. Torn.

— years of knowing I needed to do more for me, like exercise regularly, assess my eating plan or just consider what I need in any given moment, but refusing to give this any priority, not knowing how to give this priority

— years of feeling like I was one breath away from drowning in life, treading water.

Living like this is so complicated and totally not what is right for me.

Or for you.

Listening to the messages that my body is sending me and knowing intuitively what I need to do for myself at all times is much simpler and is totally what is right for me.

And for you.

Will you walk in the garden and close your eyes to appreciate the fragrance of the frangipani blossom? Does that speak directly to your senses?

I do enjoy a vase full of flowers on my table – they look beautiful and add colour to any room. I enjoy the thrill I get when I open the door to a florist with an armful of colourful blooms just for me, followed by the disappointment that floods over me when I breathe in their fragrance and there is none. The relationship with my senses ends there.

I have even bought flowers for myself on occasion, which is a lovely thing to do.

But those gestures are just that. Gestures.

I much prefer flowers in the ground, thriving in the soil. I have a rose garden outside my bedroom window. I planted *Eiffel Tower* rose bushes in this garden to remind me of my love for Paris. The way the scent of my roses wafts through my open window and fills my senses gives me a sense of wholeness and wonder.

I rejoice each summer when my frangipani

blooms – the vivid duo-colour contrast and the amazing fragrance, even more prominent when I close my eyes and engage solely with my sense of smell. I grew it from a cutting and it is growing slowly, getting a little bigger each year. Yet it always flowers and I always rejoice.

Spring and autumn are my favourite seasons both in and out of the garden. New flowers blossoming, the bees are buzzing around the place and butterflies fluttering. It is a wonderland of nature that gives me such joy.

Do you make time in your life for a garden? Do you nurture your plants? Does this give you joy?

Are you someone who curses each time you arrive home or go outdoors and see the overgrown weeds and dead plants that could not survive without water and nurturing? Do you sigh and wish you weren't so busy – shrugging your shoulders and totally missing the point that you can change your busy-ness? – that you are in control of how busy you are?

What you fill your day with is your choice, it is not something that somebody else is in control of. Whether your choices are aligned with what you need is what you need to consider more carefully.

Does your garden reflect the priority you give to self-care? Often, our home environment – the state of our home and our garden – reflects the state of our inner emotions.

I find gardening very therapeutic; when I'm weeding, trimming and nurturing, I simultaneously process the thoughts and feelings that come into my mind at the time. I process issues that I am confronted with and feel uneasy about, while I toil in the garden and often make decisions about letting go or taking action.

When I am in the garden, I am able to be with myself; to be with my thoughts, with my feelings. I am able to align with myself. What could be a higher priority than that?

For this analogy I have used the garden. This reflection is really about giving time to the things that enrich you, that make you come alive; giving time to the things that help you to be fully aligned, to be serene.

I have learned that when I am angry, frustrated and upset I have the choice to either act out, project these feelings onto something or someone else or disconnect with myself; or I can seek out things that create serenity for me, things that ground me and create a stable space

for me to process why I am feeling that way,
why I am having that reaction.

Do you glory in the feel of the sun on your face?
Does this give you hope and an urge to dance? Does
the beauty of the sunrise stop your mind?

I have spent most of my life dressing co-dependently. I seek an image that does not attract attention to my physical body. I learned at a very young age that being pretty can attract the attention of pedophiles. I learned the connection between choosing clothing and appearing invisible. I grew up with a shame-based identity as a result of verbal and sexual abuse.

When I was in my twenties, I was crossing the Highway, having just got off the bus from work. As I waited in the middle of the highway, watching the oncoming traffic for when it was safe for me to continue across, a man driving a truck tooted at me. I thought nothing of this; until ten minutes later, he was knocking at my door. *"Hi, I saw you on the highway, you looked so beautiful, I knocked on every door until I found you."*

He came again very early the next morning

and forced his way into my house when I opened the door to his knock, more asleep than awake. This became a year-long saga that ended up with the man being charged with aggravated assault and found guilty in a court of law.

A year-long saga that continues to traumatise me many years later. I no longer walk alone as I do not feel safe. I find it difficult to dress without thinking of how my outfit may attract unwanted attention.

This experience gives me insight into how life experiences can affect how we choose to dress.

Of course, this is only one of the worms in this particular can.

I see so many people having surgical procedures to maintain an image of youth

— fighting against the aging process or in pursuit of perfection as they see themselves as imperfect

— unable to love themselves in their natural state

— not able to love the laughter lines or the changes in their appearance that come with age

— seeking to be their definition of beauty

— hoping that achieving this perfection will bring them happiness.

To me, beauty radiates from within and is natural. Beauty is the curve in your neck. Beauty is your vulnerability. Kindness in your eyes. Love in your voice.

Beauty is you comforting an upset child.

Beauty is taking in a stray kitten that would not live if you did not.

Beauty is being with yourself for as long as it takes.

Beauty is being with another for as long as it takes.

I guess I have no qualms about any process that will make me less noticeable, aging included. I seek to be invisible.

Different sides of the same coin? I think so.

This is an area of dysfunction I am currently working through because I would like to feel less shame and have the freedom to choose to dress however I would like to, with the objective to feel good about myself and nothing else.

I live in a country – Australia - that has a lot of sunshine all year round, which means most of the population has a tan to some degree, not to mention a very high incident of skin cancer.

Some people have an intentional goal of achieving a deep and rich tan to tie in with the image they are aiming for, regardless of the risk to their skin.

From the age of eighteen until I became a mother, I used to prioritise time for laying in the sun and working on my tan. I would lather myself with coconut oil and literally bake my skin. I look back on that time and know it was madness. Yet the younger me would not have heeded any warning.

Once I became a parent and I became conscious of protecting the alabaster skin of my children, I made the decision to keep my skin out of the sun, or at least protect my skin better than I had previously. Becoming a parent made me realise I wanted to be around to share my children's lives, to be a part of their journey.

I became less vain for a variety of reasons: lack of time; less disposable income; experiencing a love that helped me to realise what was important in this life. And eventually, self-love.

I now seek the sunshine, to feel the touch of the sun on my skin, nothing more. I turn my face to the sun, close my eyes and just *be*. Delicious!

Whenever I witness a sunrise or a sunset, I am astounded every time, as if it were my first.

Watching the colour-palette of the sky change as the sun emerges or subsides truly stops all thought in my mind and I am completely immersed in that experience. Completely. And when the sun sinks into the ocean (horizon) I feel a sigh.

These are the moments I live for. They have nothing to do with how I look; nothing to do with my image and yet they radiate out of me.

These moments have everything to do with my heart and my soul.

Can you feel your heartbeat when your fingers are entwined in mine; does this give you the sense that you are home?

Home. The state of being when my thoughts are aligned with my actions, when my vibration is humming and I feel completely at ease in my own skin, where I feel no emotional or energy blockages, where I am completely accepting of myself. This is home. Home is a sacred place that I cherish.

I no longer wear jewelry as a rule. I do not like the way jewelry makes me feel like my energy flow is restricted. I do not like the weight of jewelry on my skin. On a very rare occasion I will wear a bangle or a ring, or I will change my ear-rings. But I usually only wear ear-rings, the same ones most of the time.

I like to receive gifts, even though I prefer to give. Since being diagnosed with *Waldenstrom's Macroglobulinaemia*, I have learned to receive with gratitude and humbleness, not necessarily the giving of material gifts, but more the gifts of compassion and understanding; of the hugs I receive just at the moment that I may stumble, the gift of someone else's time, compassion and an act of kindness

— the gift of a warm cup of coffee placed in my hand when I am numb

— the healing touch of a volunteer with just one intention: to leave me better off than when they found me.

I cannot be with someone who would shower me with gifts, but gave no priority to holding my hand.

I cannot be with someone who makes me feel that I am temporary.

I cannot be a person who would rather give myself a token gift than to be with myself.

I want to live my life in sync with the beat of my heart.

I understand that my home is within, not the four walls and roof under which I sleep.

When I celebrated my 21st birthday, my father was to bring along the birthday cake. The party was a river cruise aboard a river boat and my dad simply did not show up. I was certainly put out that I didn't have a birthday cake, but I was completely shattered by the fact that my dad did not come to celebrate my birthday with me. He never apologised or acknowledged his absence. I nursed that emotional pain for many years, an emotional block I carried around with me for a long, long time.

Ironically, I sit outside my father's hospital room at this very moment. He is experiencing his final sunset and growing his angel wings. Eighty-one years of age. I no longer struggle to let go of the things that have upset me. I listen to the sound of his breath entering and leaving his body and this brings me great comfort. It is profoundly intimate to be with my dad in his final hours when we both know that he is dying and that the words we exchange and the time we share will be the last.

Each year my children ask me if there is anything in particular I would like for my birthday or for Christmas and I really do give this thought. Every time my heart's response is that the only thing I want is to be with them on these occasions; the joy of having them with me is all my heart calls for.

This Christmas just past, my daughter was really upset because she had ordered my gift via her girlfriend who would not give her clear information about whether this gift would arrive in time. It turned out that it did not. I asked my daughter if she could let go of her hurt and the disappointment of not being able to give her gift to me because the thing that was most important to me was that I was with her in each moment. If she was upset about the gift not arriving, something that was now in the past and over which she had no control, then she was not present and I could sense her absence.

Life is the most precious thing. Life is the title of the story. Living is the story.

That my heart is beating and I am alive and that my children – the greatest loves of my life – are alive and with me is what is most important to me.

That the people who have taken a part of me and given a part of themselves to me are part of my story, is the solution to the mystery of my life.

For many years I was seeking something greater than myself. The elusive "it" that I could never quite manage to find.

Now I know.

Do you long for that moment when there is only your heartbeat and mine and you know you have found your other half?

According to Greek mythology, humans were originally created with four arms, four legs and a head with two faces. Fearing their power, Zeus split them into two separate parts, condemning them to spend their lives in search of their other halves.

The romantic in me loves this theory.

I have thought I had found my other half twice in my life. The latest being in the summer of 2018 only to have him shut me out and break my heart. I struggled with letting him go, to feel whole without him in my life. How did I know he was my soul mate and not just a lover? You do not get to choose a soul mate. I often call out to him across time and he no longer answers me.

I have tried to love again, but it has not worked out for me. I have not felt that soul connection and I knew it was not what I wanted or what I needed, that it could not fulfil me or sustain me.

Yet I yearn for the person that I am in relationship – shared looks that speak loudly without saying a word – touches in passing that are promises for later – frozen moments in time like photos imprinted on my mind – a heart connection that touches my soul. I see a field of flowers where there is an empty paddock.

Above all else, I nurture the relationship that I have with myself. I know with certainty that it is from this relationship that all love flows.

I go often to the place of stillness, where there is only my heartbeat and my love for me. The place where I know I am magical and that I am whole and worthy of everything wondrous.

All of my life experiences, bringing me to that moment, I am able to feel peace and contentment and I have an absolute knowing that everything is as it should be.

Living authentically has required that I break lifelong patterns and a whole lot of letting go; letting go of the familiar, letting go of fear.

Un-becoming.

I have learned the beauty of an emotional mess; that vulnerability is the most intimate gift you can give to yourself or another.

Those are huge things, right? It really does take courage to come out into the open with your vulnerability exposed and to stay there without covering up.

At some stage, I am not sure when exactly, it became more second nature than a conscious effort. I still have situations where I need to walk myself through it, however, walk through it I do.

Heart open.

Authentic.

I have been seeing a wonderful man for a while and that relationship is teaching me a lot about myself and I have been confronted with my insecurities and unhealthy, conditioned beliefs about my sexuality. I have had anger and acted out of this place, ended things only to process my fear and reach out to him again and again. I am not sure whether it is falling off the wagon or climbing back onto the wagon. Sadly, recently, he ended our relationship, just after my second round of chemotherapy / immunotherapy started. I am still putting back the pieces, however, with strong resolve to move forward with my life, my heart open and living each day to its greatest potential.

I am learning to recognise how rejection and

abandonment trigger childhood trauma memories and I see the opportunity for me to accept that part of me and to love her and to be there for her always.

I do not have a genuine wish to harm another person as I believe that doing so harms me and sends out harmful energy into the world. Each time I ended things, I felt loss and I felt afraid for what life would be like for me without this person in it – I still do.

I have learned to take those emotions by the hand and comfort them for as long as it takes.

I have learned that it is okay to cry when I am sad, that is not weakness. Although rarely can I cry unless I am alone.

I have learned that fear is necessary for me to know myself truly, but it has no power over me unless I relinquish.

I have learned that anger tells me when I don't like something but is not a weapon to be used against myself or others.

I have learned that the only lasting, loving relationship that I am able to have from the day I am born until the day that I die, is that with myself, whether or not that makes me whole.

*Can you hear me calling for you in the silence;
will you come to me without thinking about what
time you must get up for work?*

I find it really difficult to ask for help when
I need it. I spent many years being the rock for
other people in my life as well as being my own
rock. Self-reliance 101.

When I was a child, if I needed to ask
something or I couldn't do a task properly, I
was terrified of the consequences. I learned
from a very young age to rely only on myself, a
self-reliance instilled in me so deeply that I find
it very difficult to receive help to this very day.

I began to believe it was a sign of weakness
to ask for help and I knew absolutely it was not
safe. I became totally self-sufficient.

I had very little trust in other people; that
they would help me with no strings attached.

Childhood trauma led me to believe that
people could not be trusted and the only time I
felt safe was when I was alone.

I had a habit of working out the worst

outcome in any given situation and expecting that outcome. That way I figured I could only be pleasantly surprised if things worked out better than the worst outcome.

I recall Christmas time when I was young. My dad was a thoroughbred race horse trainer and we would wait for him to finish work in the stables so we could open our Christmas gifts. It seemed he would find anything to do in the stables to avoid coming for Christmas. It felt like an eternity to me and it really took the joy out of Christmas for me as a child. I continue to struggle at Christmas.

I've experienced exhausting days after being up all night with my sick child; after comforting my child after a bad dream or because anxiety kept me awake. I will do whatever it takes to help myself or those I love to get through, with no thought for time or what I have to do the next day.

When I was married, and raising small children, my then-husband would not get up to a sick child and he would not hear me crying through the night if I was sad. He often told me he had to get up early which is why he did not do those things.

He never saw the drop of my shoulders. He

never saw that my eyes were brimming with tears. He did not notice that I was quiet. As long as the house was clean and the children were looked after, he did not notice me at all.

The lack of these things throughout most of my life has helped me to come to the realisation that this missing part of me, the missing thing in my life, has been my ability to love myself enough to be there for as long as it takes and as often as needed; to accept my struggle as a beautiful thing that with self-care and self-support my beautiful little girl will emerge and shine.

After a cancer diagnosis, I have learned to both ask for help and to accept help. I have learned to receive with grace and without guilt. Receiving has softened me immensely. I realise how much asking for help is an act of self-love. No more insisting on doing everything myself – an unhealthy form of martyrdom.

I recently completed six cycles of chemotherapy and immunotherapy to treat the cancer, because my body had stopped producing enough blood. I was terrified when I was faced with making this decision. Since diagnosis, the monster under my bed has been the possibility of chemotherapy. Something which I believed could end my life. I was very overwhelmed and struggling to know what to do next. A friend approached me and asked if I would accept her help to co-ordinate support people and anything else that I may need throughout the treatment. I said a big fat YES! I had a team of people willing to help in various ways and I never went to any of the treatments alone. This made such a difference to how I coped with the treatment over six months. Knowing that I had a team of support made such a difference.

After diagnosis, I developed severe anxiety and post-traumatic stress disorder. I struggled with this for eighteen months or so before I conceded that I needed help, including medication and therapy. During that eighteen months I barely slept, resorting to medication to help me to sleep. I was so ashamed about my mental health that I stopped going to social events and spent most of my time either walking or at home. My world became very small, as I avoided anything that would trigger me. It was a living hell. When I felt I was on the verge of a breakdown, I asked my doctor for help.

The help I received and continue to receive

literally saved me.

Identifying that I needed help is a part of being with myself for as long as it takes. It has been a long mental health journey, albeit one of wonderful self-discovery.

Are you mesmerised by the curve of my neck and the smile in my eyes? Do you see the bee on the rosebud as a wondrous thing?

Do you see what is right in front of your eyes? Are you too caught up in your thoughts to see what is right in front of your eyes? Are you too busy?

Are you desensitised to being in the moment, completely?

Would you crush a field of sunflowers, just to get to the other side? Would you even notice?

I have been all of those things, with the exception of crushing flowers. I would go the long way around. Every time.

I remember falling into a heap of human jelly when I heard the words *you have cancer,* and thinking I would not function ever again. I had all these tentacles of emotion that were my nerve endings reaching out desperately to find something to hold onto to. Seeking security.

I was absolutely terrified.

I was a pile of rubble and human tissue with

a screaming mind that was stuck on play.

All I could do was observe myself.

It turns out that observation was how I began to put myself together; how I began to rebuild, to recover.

A lifetime of not seeing what was in front of my eyes.

A lifetime of being too caught up in my thoughts.

A lifetime of being too busy.

A lifetime of being completely desensitised, until I could no longer live like that.

Why? I had stopped feeling. I was living a numb existence. What I have learned is that you cannot choose what you feel. You either feel everything or you feel nothing. To cope with what was happening when I was young, I learned to dissociate and become numb.

I know now that I want to feel everything, rather than have an absence of love and joy. I also know that I am able to accept situations that cause me pain and sadness and to sit with myself and allow those feelings to "be", knowing that I am safe to do so.

Can you see the future and the past when you look into my eyes? Can you see my mood in the way I hold my shoulders?

Every day we take in massive amounts of data and information received visually, verbally and through smell and taste.

When I was raising my children, I was literally overloaded with information from the time I opened my eyes until I closed them, sometimes even after I closed them, as my mind would not turn off – particularly when I had spent the day preparing for an exam. My mind would keep going over the information no matter how much I tried to sleep – listening to the children when they asked me something, which was constant when they weren't at school, helping with homework, reading stories; trying to co-ordinate our busy schedules of work, school, extra-curricular activities, sport and the kids' after school employment, meant that my mind was processing information all of the time.

Then throw in undergraduate university study toward a business degree, followed by a TAFE Diploma and heavy involvement in primary school P&C Association and Secretary of the Basketball Association.

When anxiety was at its peak, my mind simply could not stop, finding anything to worry about. I had months of living in an extremely stressed condition and on very little sleep, before succumbing to medication.

No longer working means I have time to work out what is really important to me. It means I have time to notice things I did not notice before. I have time for me and time to invest in my health and well-being.

I realise that I filled my life to the brim, to distract my thoughts, to dull out my soul's calling, to seek approval from others that I was a wonderful mother and a capable woman.

No distractions now. Living my best life is about being fully present in each moment, showing up for myself always and focusing only on what is best for me. It is such a simple existence and my vibration is so smooth and constant.

Having finished treatment a week ago, I am able to rest to the extent that my body needs it.

No soldiering on for me. There is no reward for ignoring your body's needs. It is self-punishment, nothing less.

Being able to be myself in each moment; accepting my past and trusting that 'now' will take care of my future means that I feel completely safe. When I am alone, this is a lot easier than when I am with someone, particularly if I am in a relationship. I know that I want to be authentic, yet I find myself in protection mode, keeping my past in a dark corner and uncertain of my future. There is learning and growth to do. Being able to sit with myself is the key to this growth.

Close friendships are the same. I know my tribe because I feel whole around them. If I am unable to feel safe around a person, I no longer invest in that relationship. Feeling safe means I am able to be completely authentic, to stand in my truth, and feel loved and accepted.

Would you be willing to go against what is right for you to be my friend or will you always stay true to your values and beliefs even if that means hurting my feelings?

Over my lifetime, I have often gone against my beliefs and values to keep the peace in a relationship. I have swallowed my words when I have strongly disagreed with what is happening, to avoid conflict. I still do — sometimes. If I have nothing to say, it is a good indication that I do not like the situation. It was not until I was in my thirties that I started to realise what my values and belief systems were; to realise what I felt strongly about; to realise what virtues were important to me. The impact on my soul every time I accepted behaviour that went against everything I believe, hurt me to my core.

To me, my values and beliefs are the promises I make to myself. They are integral to my boundaries — both in how I treat others and how others treat me. When those values and beliefs are compromised, I feel a deep sense of self-betrayal, abandonment, anxiety and sadness because I know I am not standing in my truth; I am not being authentic; I am not being real.

This issue lies at the centre of co-dependency: choosing to behave in a way that goes against your beliefs and values to avoid conflict or to keep another person happy.

Since cancer diagnosis I have been seeking out my truth and choosing to live authentically so that I may live my best life, so that I may live fully.

Living my best life is nothing to do with dining in the finest restaurants, living in a flash house, or having a wardrobe full of designer clothes and shoes. It has everything to do with honouring myself in everything I do and always acting in accordance with my own integrity – my values and beliefs.

There is no reason good enough to compromise my values and beliefs, my code of truth.

My relationship with myself is the most important relationship I have and will always come before any other relationship.

Living by my code of truth is no simple task.

A lot of the people I know and love do not respond kindly to this change in me. Going from a people-pleaser to someone who stands firmly in their own truth has caused some conflict. I have ended some significant relationships rather than compromise my code of truth.

I have endured pain and loss because I have ended relationships. There have been lots of tears. But I have not lost my sense of self. I have not felt abandoned or betrayed. I have not felt disempowered or co-dependent. I have been able to stand in my integrity and truth knowing I have not abandoned myself.

I have been able to heal also. Ending relationships with people that you love deeply and are enmeshed with causes pain and trauma, particularly those relationships in which I have been co-dependent and I have abandoned my code of truth to avoid conflict and to avoid someone being disappointed in me. Those relationships either require that I continue to behave in the same way or that the other person deal with how they feel when I stand in my truth and say that I don't like certain behaviour or treatment, or the relationship cannot continue.

I have ended several relationships that were very important to me rather than compromise my code of truth – my marriage and several friendships.

I recently ended a thirty-four year friendship with someone I considered to be my best friend. She was in a marriage that created mostly negative emotions for her. This had been happening for five years. During that time, I have accepted things that go against my code of truth and this has left me feeling troubled and inauthentic. I became very aware I had entered into co-dependent behaviour with my best friend, rather than tell her that I did not like certain things.

Until recently. She got into the habit of only calling me when she was on her way to work or on her way home from work – in the car – or when her husband wasn't at home. If I called when her husband was at home, she would reject my call and message that he was there, or she would go outside and regulate the volume of her voice to ensure he could not hear her. I was very aware of this. I did not like this, at all. But I continued to accept this because I didn't want to let her down. I knew she needed to talk to someone and feel heard.

She had been having a trial separation from her husband for a couple of months. I was delighted at the time that I was no longer compromising my code of truth because I was able to call her with free-spiritedness as her husband was not living with her.

As they tried to work out whether they would stay married, they made a pact that neither of them would be on their phones while in each other's company – which resulted in me being unable to speak with my best friend on her birthday as she spent the bulk of the day with her husband. I knew this agreement they made meant that I would need to decide whether I would revert back to co-dependent behaviour to keep this friendship, or whether I would say that I no longer accept this treatment. It really was not a difficult decision because I know I want to live my best life, absolutely. I know that I want to stand in my truth at all times.

Having unknowingly chosen co-dependent behaviour most of my life, the internal struggle was real. Finding the words to tell my best friend that I did not accept that treatment and actually sending them to her was not an easy thing for me to do. But I did find the words and sent them to her. She was unable to accept my truth and said that I was treating her badly, therefore the relationship was not sustainable in the absence of co-dependency.

Perhaps in time, there will be a relationship without co-dependency. What is really important to note is that my relationship with myself is intact. There is no berating myself for not standing in my truth, there is no grief for abandoning myself in favour of another.

I now have the courage and self-love to refuse to compromise my code of truth, even if that means disappointing someone that I love.

Can I share with you my deepest secrets and fears and know that you won't use them against me?

During my marriage, after the birth of my daughter, I recalled suppressed memories of sexual abuse as a child. I spent a year or so as part of a crisis care group through an organisation for the support of sexual abuse and violence for women. This was a time of immense pain for me, as I tried to make some sort of sense out of what had happened to me as a child – things so horrible that I suppressed them until I had my own daughter. Then the memories came bubbling up and overwhelmed me. In many senses, I was emotionally crippled. At this time my husband chose to leave me, taking with him the baby seat for the car and any access I had to money, while knowing I had the sole care of our infant daughter.

To say this time was difficult is an understatement. Looking back on my life, this is one of the times I really did not think I would survive.

When a child is physically, verbally and sexually abused, trust is a major issue. The child does not develop in the way that healthy and happy children are able to. She has no sense of value or worth. I lived in great fear most of the time and developed amazing survival skills that revolved around complete lack of trust in my care-givers. I learned to analyse at a very young age and those skills have been well honed over the years.

Until these memories came simmering into my consciousness, I could not begin to heal.

I separated from my husband seven times during my marriage of seven years. I was afraid a lot of the time, raising our children and working part-time while keeping a home. He could be violent and as I still live in the home we bought together, there are holes in doors as a result of his anger erupting. I did not know that I was anxious at the time, but I could barely go to the mail box some days. My social network of friends had completely disappeared and I was isolated.

When I left my husband for the final time, I recall him saying to me that he felt he should be compensated for having to put up with my flaws and issues as a result of my childhood trauma. Of everything that I had endured through my marriage, this was one of the most hurtful things he said to me.

As I walked away from him, he also said to me that I would never find someone to love me like he did. I am pleased to say that I found someone to love me a lot more than he could – me.

Through therapy I came to understand that I have a shame-based identity. Because I had been unable to develop in a healthy way in any area, I felt shame around speaking up for myself, the way I look, my sexuality and my sensuality.

I am currently working on lessening the amount of shame I feel about myself and hope I am able to reprogram the way I identify with myself. I realise that to succeed, to progress, it is not enough to just read material. I realise I need to challenge myself to incorporate things that cause me to feel shamed into my everyday life so I can be with my feelings and reassure myself that I am lovable in those moments. This takes such courage as I am facing fear and no longer hiding from it. I am committed to no longer giving in to my insecurities. I am committed to no longer limiting myself so I will not feel a certain way.

I have come to understand that to have a healthy relationship with myself or with another, how essential it is that I can express my deepest secrets and fears safely and know that I will not turn on myself or have them held against me or thrown at me by someone I trusted enough to confide in.

To me, this truth and trust is vital.

When someone shares something with you about their life, this is personal information that comes from a vulnerable and trusting place. I know when I share something personal about myself it is usually because I need to speak about it with someone, to get it out of my body and out of my mind so I can see it differently and take steps to process my experience, with a view to deciding how best to move forward. This is a precious gift of trust.

Many times, when I have shared something of myself, the person I have entrusted with my confidence has been dismissive and invalidating, totally oblivious of the combination of trust and vulnerability that has taken place and proving untrustworthy – which has led to isolation and withdrawal. The truth is that I need connection with myself and with others. Isolation as a way of life does not serve me. It creates an even deeper lack of trust and results in my thoughts going around and around in my head.

The only way to build trust is risk your vulnerability. This is what I have discovered.

This sharing of one's truth is something completely opposite to live theatre, a good movie or a good book. It is the opposite of the escapism. It is being fully present. It is fully seeing someone.

Will you intuitively know that when I love someone I give a piece of myself to them to take as their own? And when someone I love dies, that piece of me dies with them?

I stood beside you, in the tender silence. I knew it was you, even though it didn't look like you.

They were your hands, beyond a doubt; folded peacefully on your chest, hands that had endured over your lifetime and became testament to a life of fighting and toil – a life of stroking a horse's neck, of tweaking reins; of buckling a girth; of punching holes in walls, in rage – the hands that I had held in mine in your final days.

Hands that had never before been folded peacefully on your chest.

You had your dentures in and this made your face look different; your top lip was fuller. Your chest sucked in, as though your last breath had been a desperate gasp for air before your heart stopped beating. In this moment I could sense your suffering and this distressed me.

The gold plaque on the lid of your coffin was inscribed: *Daniel Frederick Duggan 1938-2019*. It was resting against the wall, ready to be placed on your coffin when the time came for you to leave the chapel.

It was a stunning day. The sunlight spilled in through the windows and cast a soft light on your face. I stood, holding your hand and thinking how cold your fingers felt, yet comforted that I could spend this time with you, the most intimate moment I would ever share with you. It hit me then, the pure love that I have for you. I didn't know why, but I knew I would be at peace with you now after a lifetime of being at odds with you, a lifetime of suffering the trauma of a torrid childhood with you, an explosive, angry and unpredictable father; many years as an adult, suffering the pain of making poor choices through the filter of childhood trauma. It all just drifted away; vanished and left me with peace and pure love in my heart for you.

And such grief. Such loss. So many tears.

My sister knew my grief. She was there too, silently wiping away the pain that welled in her eyes and spilled down her cheeks. She knew my loss, it was her loss too.

My brother knew my grief: he was protecting us in the room, staying strong and loving us without saying a word. It was his name on the coffin lid, having been given the same name as his father.

For me, to love someone is to give a part of myself to them, to care for as their own, and for me to take a part of them to care for as my own. When that someone you love cares poorly for that part of you, it means they do not care for themselves. It does not mean they do not care for you. They are caring for that part of you, as if it were part of them.

I've learned how important self-love really is. How vital it is to nurture the relationship that I have with myself, so I can be authentic. Which means I can be completely emotionally available for all of my relationships, including with myself, including those parts of others that I love and take for my own.

I know now that my Dad did not lack love for me, he was emotionally unavailable because his relationship with himself was poor. He had little self-worth and no self-love. So, when I gave a part of me to him for him to care for as his own, that caretaking had the same capacity that he had to love himself.

I have told many people that I love them. Fortunately for them, as my relationship with myself has blossomed, so too has my love for that part of them that I care for as my own.

Yet, nothing compares to when I told my Dad that I loved him for the last time. He was dying and we talked about that. I asked him how he felt about knowing that he was dying. He shrugged his shoulders and said, "*it is what it is*". Obviously, I was struggling more with the concept of his impending death than he seemed to be. He had suffered so much. Maybe suffering simplifies the path to the afterlife.

I do not know how, but I knew it was so very important to me that my Dad knew he was loved when he was dying, that he knew he would never be forgotten; that I would remember him always. That I got to tell him this was one of the most precious gifts ever.

When my dad died and I was preparing for his funeral, my lover at that time asked me if I really wanted him to be there to hold my hand. He asked in such a way that made it clear to me he did not want to go. My answer was simple: if he did not want to go then I did not want him there. I knew then on some level the damage that caused to our future. He had no concept of love in the sense that I know love, the way that love works for me. That part of me had died when my Dad took his last breath, that as my lover, he would know he needed to be there, because I needed him to be. I also understood that funerals make him very emotional and that, like many people, he avoids situations that make him feel sad or conflicted. I know that journey only too well.

Will you lead me to the sunshine if I am living in the shade? Will you encourage me to abandon the limits that I place on myself, to lift the lid so that I can be the best version of me?

This is about leaving every person you come into contact with, better than they were before, without compromising yourself. It is about being present when you come across someone else, no matter what is going on for you. It is about fully seeing someone even if they have retreated to a safe place.

I sense a lot of emotional pain around me and also inside of me. The pain and suffering in the world is phenomenal, whether you choose to see it or not. It is there. It is not something that is conjured by negative or depressed people. It is not something that is invalidated by those people who live in denial and choose to believe that only positive thinking is allowed and anything else will not exist.

So many people do not value themselves, do not love themselves, or even like themselves.

It is not difficult to become isolated, to find yourself unbelonging and alone. I am sure we have all been there at some time in our lives. I know that I have.

If I can help someone to light a small candle when they are in their darkness, even for a moment, I am compelled to do this. The way that a candle shows the beauty of darkness, like nothing else can, is simply beautiful. Sometimes, we need a hand to take ours and lead the way.

When I hit the wall and sit with myself, in the shade, until I am spent and the storm has passed, I am able to walk outside and put my face to the sun. Most times.

I was not always able to do this and I still find it difficult sometimes. However, inevitably, I manage to make my way into the sunshine again.

Lifting the Lid, in the context of this book, means no longer suppressing past trauma and having the courage and commitment to let these memories and feelings free. No matter that they make me nauseous. No matter that they make me sad, afraid and angry beyond rage.

I recognise how vital it is to my healing and

the letting go process that I no longer keep these memories and emotions locked away inside my mind and my body.

That is what this book is about: being there for myself and for my inner child and having the same compassion toward others; realising there is nowhere more important for me to be than with myself or another when I am needed.

Everything flows from that.

Lifting the Lid is also about no longer limiting myself; no longer telling myself that my dreams are too grand or too unrealistic; not allowing my inner critic to shoot me down when I think I might like to try something new and unknown, when I might want to do something adventurous; not allowing that sadistic voice in my head to shame me when things do not work out how I expected them to.

Lifting the Lid is about being proud that I tried, even if it was not the outcome I wanted; being wise enough to know that the trying is the important thing and not the end result. The trying is what helps me to grow and to know myself.

The biggest limit I have is myself. Only in recognising this and acknowledging this can I live without a lid, without the limitations I place on myself.

Faith is believing in something that cannot be seen.

My relationships, the people I love, also incorporate the premise that I will encourage others to be the best version of themselves possible, no matter how poorly someone else may treat them; to encourage each other that the only limits we have are those we impose on ourselves; to light the candle for one another when we find ourselves in darkness.

This is how I choose to live my life.

This is how I live my best life in every given moment.

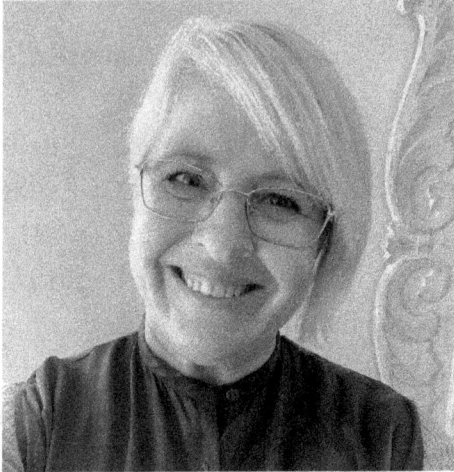

About the Author

Mandy Duggan is a published author, blogger and songwriter who lives in the south west of Western Australia. Retirement in 2015 due to a chronic health condition was life-changing and Mandy wrote her first book as a powerful healing tool for herself and readers. Mandy felt compelled to share her own story; if her journey could help just one person then it made it worthwhile. Becoming a published author has also created the opportunity for Mandy to give inspirational talks which have been an amazing experience.